BLOOD PRESSURE SOLUTION

60 Delicious Heart Healthy Recipes that will Naturally Lower High Blood Pressure and Decrease Hypertension

© Copyright 2017 by Mark Evans - All rights reserved.

The following Book is reproduced below with the goal of providing information that is as accurate and as reliable as possible. Regardless, purchasing this Book can be seen as consent to the fact that both the publisher and the author of this book are in no way experts on the topics discussed within, and that any recommendations or suggestions made herein are for entertainment purposes only. Professionals should be consulted as needed before undertaking any of the action endorsed herein.

This declaration is deemed fair and valid by both the American Bar Association and the Committee of Publishers Association and is legally binding throughout the United States.

Furthermore, the transmission, duplication or reproduction of any of the following work, including precise information, will be considered an illegal act, irrespective whether it is done electronically or in print. The legality extends to creating a secondary or tertiary copy of the work or a recorded copy and is only allowed with express written consent of the Publisher. All additional rights are reserved.

The information in the following pages is broadly considered to be a truthful and accurate account of facts, and as such any inattention, use or misuse of the information in question by the reader will render any resulting actions solely under their purview. There are no scenarios in which the publisher or the original author of this work can be in any fashion deemed liable for any hardship or damages that may befall them after undertaking information described herein.

Additionally, the information found on the following pages is intended for informational purposes only and should thus be considered, universal. As befitting its nature, the information presented is without assurance regarding its continued validity or interim quality. Trademarks that mentioned are done without written consent and can in no way be considered an endorsement from the trademark holder.

Table of Contents

Introduction 1

FREE BONUS BOOK 3

The Dangers of a Rising Blood Pressure 5

Breakfast Recipes 17

Lunch Recipes 43

Snack and Side Recipes 63

Dinner Recipes 87

Dessert Recipes 105

Conclusion 123

Thank you! 125

INTRODUCTION

Congratulations on purchasing your very own copy of *Blood Pressure Solution*. Thank you so much for doing so!

This book will discuss one of the most probable causes of death in America today: the rise of blood pressure levels. Blood pressure plays a big role in keeping our bodies at a healthy and maintained level for survival. Decreases and increases in this variable can cause major health complications down the road, but I am here to inform you that you can fix it by making small changes in your diet!

The contents of this book are filled with valuable information that will help support you in your journey of lowering your blood pressure by your next doctor appointment! You will discover that what you consume is the major cause of why your blood pressure is higher than it should be.

Each of the recipes tucked away within the chapters of this book are designed to keep you on the straight and narrow as you get your blood pressure under control, all while not sacrificing taste and satisfaction! Each recipe includes the components needs to prepare them, preparation times, nutritional facts and one of the most important factors in rising blood pressure: sodium levels.

Enjoy your journey through the pages of this recipe book as you discover more information about your health and delicious eats to try in the comfort of your own home! Good luck!

There are plenty of books regarding blood pressure on the market, so thanks again for choosing this one! Every effort was made to ensure it is full of as much useful information as possible. Please enjoy!

FREE BONUS BOOK

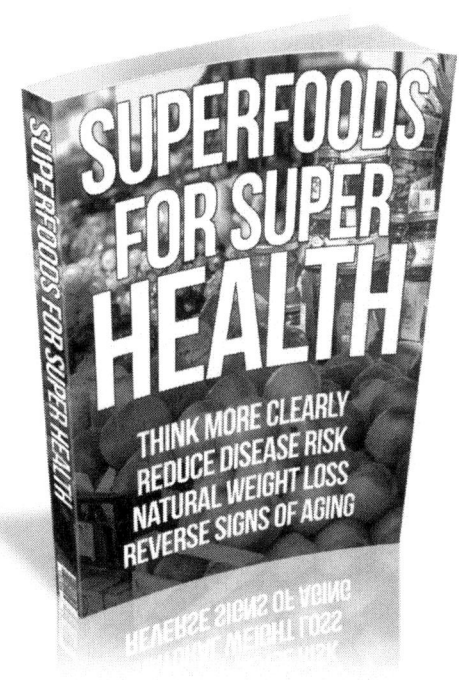

As a Thank You for purchasing this book, I would like to offer you another book as a special bonus! It is called "Super Foods For Super Health".

This comprehensive book is for those who are interested in:

- Learning more about super foods that you can easily get your hands on today.

- How to incorporate those super foods into your everyday meals.
- Nutritional benefits for each super foods
- How to improve your overall health
- How to lose weight naturally
- How to reduce disease risk
- How to reverse signs of aging
- Think more clearly
- Improving your focus
- And much more..

So if you are interested in learning more about any of the above, just go to http://bit.ly/superfoods-gift and grab your free bonus book!

THE DANGERS OF A RISING BLOOD PRESSURE

High blood pressure is something that can plague the body for many years without a person realizing it. Also referred to as hypertension, its symptoms, if left uncontrolled, can cause one to develop a disability, death by heart attack or a poor quality of the remainder of life a person has. There are many complications that come with a high blood pressure count. But fortunately, this book is here to bring to light that a change in diet alone can help to decrease your overall blood pressure immensely!

Complications of Hypertension

Destruction of the arteries

Arteries that are healthy are strong and elastic in nature. The inner lining within them is smooth so that the blood flowing through them can flow freely through them, providing vital organs and tissues within the body with oxygen and proper nutrients. Over time, hypertension increases the amount of blood flowing through your arteries. Because of this, you may have to deal with these health issues:

- *Narrowed and damaged arteries* – High blood pressure damages cells that make up the inner lining that inhibits the arteries. When fats that you consume enter into the blood stream, they have a tendency to collect in the damaged arteries, causing them to become much less elastic which results in a limit of blood flow throughout the entirety of the body.

- *Aneurysm* – A constant heightened amount of blood moving through weakened arteries can have the potential to cause enlargements within artery walls that result in the development of an aneurysm. These bad fellas can explode and result in terrible ailments that can harm your entire life, such as bleeding internally. Aneurysms develop within the arteries in the body, but they tend to be found most often right within the aorta, known as the biggest artery in our bodies.

Deterioration of the heart

Your heart is the organ responsible for getting blood to your entire body. The presence of hypertension will result in exponential damage to your heart in numerous ways, such as:

- *Heart failure* – The strain on your heart over time that is caused by hypertension will cause the muscles in your heart to weaken, causing it to not work near as efficiently as it's supposed to. Your heart will become overwhelmed, eventually wearing out and failing. Damage from heart attacks that are also caused by high blood pressure will only add to this serious issue.

- *Enlarged left heart* – The presence of hypertension forces the heart to pump harder and more often than it usually does in order to get the required blood to all areas of your body. This will cause your left ventricle of your heart become rather stiff over time, which is known as left ventricular hypertrophy. This then inhibits your ventricle's job of being able to pump blood as efficiently as it is supposed to. This condition will increase your risk of having a heart attack, congestive heart failure and even cardiac death that can arise out of nowhere rather suddenly.

- *Coronary artery disease* – This disease affects your arteries that are responsible for providing blood right to the core of your heart muscles. Arteries become narrowed over time, which does not allow blood to flow as freely as it should throughout the arteries in your body. As a result, a person with coronary artery disease can experience irregular heart rhythms, heart attack and varying degrees of chest pain.

Damage to your brain

Your brain, just like your heart, is another crucial organ within your body that heavily relies on a constant flow of nourishing blood supply in order for it to work properly. High blood pressure can cause several issues within your noggin, like:

- *Mild cognitive impairment* – This ailment is a just the stage that lies in-between understanding all the changes that happen to one's memory when natural aging occurs and the point at which those are more susceptible to developing diseases such as Alzheimer's. Like other brain ailments, it can be caused by blocked blood flow to the brain.

- *Dementia* – This is a disease that lives within the brain that impairs normal and necessary human functions such as movement, vision, memory, reasoning, speaking, and thinking. There are a few causes that result in dementia. Vascular dementia is a result of the narrowing of arteries and the blockage within them that keeps an adequate blood supply from flowing to the brain.

- *Stroke* – Strokes happen when part of the brain becomes deprived of nutrients and oxygen, which results in the death of brain cells. High blood pressure that is uncontrolled can lead to a stroke because it damages and majorly weakens the blood vessels in your brain, resulting in them becoming narrowed, rupturing and leaking. Hypertension is also the culprit behind the development of blood clots within the arteries that directly trail the way to the brain, blocking proper blood flow and potentially causing someone to have a stroke.

- *Transient ischemic attack* – Also referred to as a mini-stroke, these attacks are very brief, due to a disruption of blood flow to the brain. It is a direct cause as a result of atherosclerosis (blood clot) which can develop from having high blood pressure. IF you have one of these attacks, you should view it as a big red flag that you may be at major risk for experiencing a full-blown stroke later down the road.

Damage to your kidneys

Your kidneys are the organ in the body that filters out other fluids that are excess and other wastes from your blood. This process is dependent on having healthy blood vessels. The presence of hypertension will lead to these vital blood vessels becoming damaged, which can then result in you developing several forms of kidney disease. The damage has the potential to be much worse in those with diabetes.

- *Kidney failure* – High blood pressure takes the gold as being one of the most popular causes for the result of kidney failure. Hypertension can damage not only the larger arteries that lead to your kidneys but also the tiny blood vessels that live within your kidneys as well. Both are crucial to a thriving life. Damage to either of these can cause your kidneys to not be fully capable of filtering waste from your body. This puts the body at risk, for wastes accumulate over time and you may have to undergo dialysis or kidney transplant.

- *Kidney scarring* – Also known as glomerulosclerosis, kidney scarring is a type of kidney damage that occurs to the glomeruli, which are mini clusters made if vessels living within your kidneys that are responsible for filtering fluids and wastes from your blood. This can leave your kidneys with the lack of capability to filter wastes effectively, which can lead to kidney failure.

- *Kidney artery aneurysm* – Aneurysms are bulges that live within the walls of vessels that occur over time. This particular type of aneurysms takes place in the artery that leads to your kidneys. High blood pressure, over time, will weaken this artery and cause sections to become enlarged and form bulges. Aneurysms can rupture and threaten the life of those who have them with internal bleeding.

Disturbances of the eyes

There are many tiny and very intricate blood vessels that provide necessary blood to that of your eyes. Just like all vessels within the body, they have the potential to become damaged over time, especially if the presence of high blood pressure wreaks havoc on your body.

- *Eye blood vessel damage* – Also referred to as retinopathy, it is caused directly by hypertension damaged the blood vessels that supply your retinas with blood. This can cause conditions like bleeding of eyes, blurred vision and at the very worst, complete vision loss. If one has diabetes and hypertension, they are at a much greater risk of developing these conditions.

- *Buildup of fluid underneath the retina(s)* – Also known as choroidopathy, this occurs when the buildup of fluid happens underneath your retina(s) due to a blood vessel (or blood vessels) that may have burst and are leaking under the retina itself. This condition can result in a major distortion of vision and even has the potential to scar your eyes, which can lead to impaired vision.

- *Nerve damage* – Also referred to as optic neuropathy, this condition results from a blockage in blood flow that damages the optic nerve. It is responsible for killing off nerve cells within the eyes, which can result in bleeding in the eyes and potential for vision loss.

Sexual dysfunction

Although ailments such as erectile dysfunction and other such medical conditions that inhibit proper sexual functions can occur as a result of aging, the presence of high blood pressure can drastically increase the likelihood of developing these sorts of conditions. Over time, hypertension damages the lining of the vessels within these areas of your body, which will mean less blood flow to the penis and vagina, which leads to the incapability of maintaining an erection and a decreased desire in sexual intercourse. Women can also have vaginal dryness and difficulty achieving orgasms.

Bone Loss

High blood pressure has the potential to increase calcium amounts and deposits within the urine. With this major decrease of calcium from the body, these are a direct result of a loss of overall bone density which can lead to breaking more bones. The risks of osteoporosis are seen more often in women.

Trouble Sleeping

With those with high blood pressure issues, a condition known as obstructive sleep apnea can occur. This condition causes the relaxation of your throat muscles, which can lead to excessive snoring. While it has been shown that hypertension itself can directly trigger sleep apnea, sleep deprivation as a result of this condition also can be a trigger as well.

Symptoms of High Blood Pressure

Hypertension can at times be hard to detect because many people live for a long time with little to no symptoms or warning signs. This means that people do not feel like they need to go to the doctor and get anything checked out, which is why so many seemingly healthy individuals suffer from the long-term effects of hypertension later on. It is important to not take these symptoms of hypertension lightly:

- Shortness of breath
- Dizziness
- Blurred vision
- Headache

Things that Raise your Blood Pressure

High blood pressure is determined by a set of numbers; the first number is 140 or higher or if the second number is 90 or higher. There are many circumstances that physicians don't know what directly causes hypertension. It is said that family history, your age and your race all have the potential to play a factor. But these things are proven to be direct causes in the development of high blood pressure:

- *Too much salt* – Sodium is known for raising your blood pressure because it plays a major role in the narrowing of your vessels within your body that enables your body to hold on to more fluid. It is best to limit the amount of salt you consume. Alongside this rule, you need to eat plenty of potassium so that you have a fighting chance to successfully balance your sodium levels and keep high blood pressure at bay.

- *Lack of exercise* - When you spend most of your time on the couch binge watching Orange is the New Black and other shows all day; you are putting yourself in danger of a rising heart rate, which makes the heart work much harder than it needs to. But during the course of the exercise, hormones in the body relax your blood vessels and help to lower blood pressure levels.

- *Being overweight* – When you weight goes up, so does the amount of blood you need to flow to the growing portions of your body. This puts more strain directly on your heart which results in your blood vessels picking up the slack. This is why a good balance of physical activity and a healthy diet are so vital to keeping your hypertension at bay.

- *Tobacco use* – Smoking cigarettes and chewing tobacco both raise your blood pressure levels. Chemicals within these products damage your vessels which then narrows them, leading them to develop hypertension.

- *Alcohol use* – Consuming alcohol heavily on a regular basis can majorly damage your heart muscles. This is why you should limit your alcohol intake.

- *Stress* – Large amounts of stress or chronic stress can cause issues with blood pressure. It leads to starting bad habits such as smoking and drinking which as you have read, are neither the best at keeping your blood pressure levels low.

As you have read, having high blood pressure has no perks! Whether you are dedicated to living a healthier lifestyle to avoid these health issues caused by hypertension later on, or you are already struggling with problems because of your blood pressure levels, the remainder of this book is filled with recipes that will aid you in your mission to lower those threatening levels! There is no need for your taste buds to suffer in order for you to be a healthier individual! That's dive into the wide array of delicious recipes, shall we?

BREAKFAST RECIPES

DURING THE COURSE OF THE NIGHT CHIA OATMEAL

Preparation time: 5 min.
Complete time: 8 hours – During the course of the night
Calories 289 – Carbs 23g – Sodium 3g – Fat 9g

What's in it:

- ¼ tsp. nutmeg
- ¼ tsp. ground ginger
- ¼ tsp. vanilla extract
- ¼ tsp. cinnamon
- ¼ tsp. ground cardamom
- 2 tbsp. shredded coconut
- 2 tbsp. chia seeds
- 1 C. coconut almond milk
- 1 C. oats

How it's made:

- Combine all components in a medium sized bowl. Top the bowl with wrap, preferably plastic.

- Frost for 8 hours or during the course of the night. (It is much better during the course of the night!)

Sarah's Easy Homemade Applesauce

Preparation time: Ten to fifteen min.
Complete time: An hour
Calories 309 – Carbs 12g – Sodium 2.5g – Fat 11g

What's in it:

- ½ tsp. ground cinnamon
- ¼ C. white sugar
- ¾ C. water
- 4 apples - peeled, cored and chopped

How it's made:

- Mix together all components in a saucepan.
- Cook covered over intermediate to immense warmth 15 into 20 min. until apples become tender.
- Let apples sit and cool and proceed to mash with a potato masher or fork.

EGG SCRAMBLE

Preparation time: 15 min.
Complete time: 40 min.
Calories 270 – Carbs 12g – Sodium 3g – Fat 11.2g

What's in it:

- ¼ C. cheddar cheese, shredded
- A sprinkle of hot pepper sauce
- Ground cayenne
- Pepper and salt
- 2 seeded and chopped tomatoes
- 4 beaten eggs
- ½ C. freshly chopped spinach
- 2 cloves of garlic, chopped
- 1 chopped onion
- 1 peeled potato

How it's made:

- Get out a small pot. Put water in it with a few dashes of salt and heat to boiling point.
- Pour in the potato and cook for 15 min. until it is tenderized yet still firm. Remove liquid, let it cool and cut up potato.
- Sauté garlic and onion in a skillet over intermediate to immense warmth.
- Then, proceed to add in spinach, cooking it until it's wilted, around 2 min.

- Decrease your heat to medium and put in eggs. Cook for 2 min. until the bottom is set.
- Mix in tomatoes and potatoes, sprinkling with salt, pepper, and cayenne as desired. Add in hot sauce as well.
- Stir mixture occasionally until the eggs are set.
- Sprinkle your scrambled eggs with grated cheese. Serve warm!

BEER BATTER CREPES

Preparation time: 5 min.
Complete time: 10-15 min.
Calories 302 – Carbs 9g – Sodium 2.2g – Fat 9g

What's in it:

- 2 tbsp. butter
- 2 tbsp. vegetable oil
- A pinch of salt
- 1 ¾ C. regular white flour
- 1 C. beer
- 1 C. milk
- 3 lightly beaten eggs

How it's made:

- Whisk beer, eggs, and milk.
- Then gradually mix in the flour.
- Pour in salt and oil, then combine mixture rapidly three to five min., so everything is well mixed. Allow the batter sit for at least 1 hour.
- Over intermediate to immense warmth, heat a 10" skillet. Brush with butter.
- Once skillet is hot but not yet smoking, pour one-third of a cup of the mixture into the central area of cooking pan you are using, ensuring batter covers the entirety of the

bottom of your skillet. Make sure to pour out the excess batter before continuing to cook.
- Cook crepe 1 to 2 min. until it becomes golden in color.
- Then, flip it over and cook other side for 30 seconds.
- Put on a plate covered in foil to ensure they are kept toasty as you continue cooking the remaining crepes.
- Continue above process until batter is all used.
- Fill with fruit, veggies or anything else you desire!

Sausage Egg Muffins

Preparation time: 10 to 15 min.
Complete time: 30 to 40 min.
Calories 299 – Carbs 11g – Sodium 5g – Fat 14g

What's in it:

- Pepper and salt
- 1 tsp. garlic powder
- 1 chopped onion
- ½ can of chopped green chili peppers
- 12 beaten eggs
- ½ pound low-sodium ground sausage

How it's made:

- Ensure that your oven is preheated to 350 degrees.
- Lightly grease some muffin cups or a muffin tin.
- In a deep skillet on intermediate to immense warmth, place sausage and cook until browned. Remove liquid and then set to the side.
- Combine all the components and sausage in a large bowl until well mixed.
- Spoon ¼ cup of the mixture into each of the muffin cups.

- Bake 15 to 20 min. until the egg has set and a toothpick put into the middle of muffins turns out with no more batter upon it.

ULTIMATE IRRESISTIBLE GRANOLA

Preparation time: 10 min.
Complete time: 30 min.
Calories 312 – Carbs 11g – Sodium 2g – Fat 8g

What's in it:

- 1 C. dried cranberries
- 1 C. raisins
- 1 ½ C. honey
- 1 C. canola oil
- 1 C. unsalted sunflower seeds
- 2 C. coconut, shredded
- 1 C. wheat germ
- 1 C. sesame seeds
- 1 C. pecans cut up
- 1 C. walnuts cut up
- 1 C. blanched slivered almonds
- 5 C. rolled oats

How it's made:

- Ensure oven is preheated to 325 degrees.
- Mix together sunflower seeds, coconut, wheat germ, sesame seeds, pecans, walnuts, almonds and oats in a bowl.
- Over intermediate to immense warmth, stir together honey and oil in a pan. Cook until blended.

- Pour honey batter over oat mixture and stir up thoroughly.
- Put batter out on 2 cookie sheets.
- Back each for 20 min. until oats and nuts are toasted.
- Once it comes out of the oven, stir in cranberries and raisins.
- Let cook and stir again in order to break up large clusters.
- Store in airtight container for 2 weeks. Enjoy!

Banana Bran Muffins

Preparation time: 20 min.
Complete time: 45 min.
Calories 256 – Carbs 17g – Sodium 4g – Fat 8.9g

What's in it:

- ¼ tsp. salt
- ½ tsp. cinnamon
- ½ tsp. baking soda
- 1 ½ tsp. baking powder
- ¾ C. regular white flour
- 1 C. whole wheat flour
- 1 tsp. vanilla extract
- ¼ C. canola oil
- 1 C. unprocessed wheat bran
- 1 C. buttermilk
- 1 C. mashed ripe bananas
- 2/3 C. packed light brown sugar
- ½ C. chocolate chips (optional)
- 1/3 C. chopped walnuts (optional)

How it's made:

- Ensure your oven is preheated until it reaches 400 degrees.
- Grease up your muffin cups or a muffin tin with greasing medium of choice.

- Mix brown sugar and eggs together, then adding in buttermilk, bananas, wheat bran, vanilla, and oil.
- In another vessel that is bowl shaped, mix together salt, cinnamon, baking soda, baking powder, and flours until combined.
- Create a divot in your dry ingredient mixture and add in wet components, stirring until mixed and smooth. Stir in chocolate chips if you have decided to use them.
- Spoon batter into muffin tins (will be full) and top with walnuts.
- Bake 15 to 25 min. until muffins are visibly golden and when you put a finger gently among the top it springs back at you.
- Allow to sit 5 min., undo edges with a butter knife and set the muffin on a rack made of wire to let cool for a few more min. before you eat. Yum!

Wake Up Smoothie

Preparation Time: 5 min.
Calories 139 – Carbs 28g – Sodium 10g – Fat 2g

What's in it:

- 1 tbsp. Splenda
- ½ C. low-fat tofu or low-fat plain yogurt
- 1 ¼ C. frozen berries of choice
- 1 banana
- 1 ¼ C. orange juice (recommended: calcium-fortified)

How it's made:

- Combine all components until smooth and creamy in a blender.
- Serve right away as a great breakfast treat to start off your day right!

CINNAMON BAKE DONUTS

Preparation time: 15 min.
Complete time: 35 min.
Calories 210 – Carbs 13g – Sodium 5g – Fat 9g

What's in it:

- 2 tsp. pure vanilla extract
- 2 tbsp. unsalted butter, melted
- 1 ¼ C. whole milk
- 1 large lightly beaten egg
- ½ tsp. salt
- ½ tsp. nutmeg
- 1 tsp. cinnamon
- 2 tsp. baking powder
- 1 ½ C. sugar
- Spray for greasing

Topping:

- ½ tsp. ground cinnamon
- ½ C. sugar
- 8 tbsp. unsalted butter

How it's made:

- Ensure oven is preheated to 350 degrees. Sprays a couple of donut pans well with greasing medium of choice.

- Sift salt, nutmeg, cinnamon, baking powder, sugar, and flour together.
- In a small bowl, stir vanilla, melted butter and egg together well.
- Pour and mix in wet mixture into dry components and combine.
- Pour your mixture into baking pans, filling each a bit more than ¾ of the way full.
- Bake 17 min., until a toothpick turns out with no batter on it.
- Let cool for at least 5 min., then put donuts on top of a sheet pan.
- *For topping:* Within a sauté pan, melt your butter. Mix together cinnamon and sugar. Set to the side for a minute.
- Dip each donut in the butter and proceed to emerge each one in cinnamon-sugar. You can sugar up one or both sides. Indulge!

French Toast

Preparation time: 20 min.
Complete time: 30 min.
Calories 260 – Carbs 20g – Sodium 11g – Fat 9.8g

What's in it:

- ½ C. warmed maple syrup
- 8 slices of white, brioche or challah bread
- ½ tsp. vanilla extract
- ¼ C. milk
- 4 eggs
- 4 tbsp. butter
- 2 tbsp. sugar
- ¼ tsp. nutmeg
- 1 tsp. ground cinnamon

How it's made:

- Combine sugar, nutmeg, and cinnamon. Set to the side.
- In a pan over intermediate to immense warmth, melt butter.
- Whisk cinnamon mixture, vanilla, milk, and eggs together and pour into a shallow container.
- Dip bread in egg mixture.
- Fry slices of bread until they are a light golden brown hue.
- Eat with warm maple syrup.

BREAKFAST POWER BALLS

Preparation time: 20 min.
Complete time: 1 hour and 20 min.
Calories 157 – Carbs 11g – Sodium 6g – Fat 19g

What's in it:

- 2 tbsp. flax seed
- ½ C. unsalted sunflower seeds
- ½ C. dried cranberries
- ½ C. mini chocolate chips
- ½ C. raw honey
- 1 C. extra-crunchy peanut butter
- 2 C. rolled oats

How it's made:

- Pulse together flax seeds, sunflower seeds, cranberries, chocolate chips, honey, peanut butter and oats in a food processor until combined. Cover and Frost for 30 min.
- With waxed paper, line a baking sheet. Form balls from the mixture and place them on the sheet. Frost for 30 min. before consuming.

Frozen Fruit Cups

Complete time: 10 min.
Calories 123 – Carbs 5g – Sodium 2g – Fat 5g

What's in it:

- 1/3 C. lemon juice
- 1 small can of frozen pineapple-orange juice concentrate (thawed)
- 6 chopped bananas
- 1 can fruit cocktail (liquid removed)
- 2 cans crushed pineapple (liquid removed)
- 2 cans mandarin oranges (liquid removed)
- 4 C. frozen peaches (thawed and chopped)

How it's made:

- Mix all components of the recipe together in a bowl until combined.
- Place fruit mixture into plastic disposable cups, covering with plastic wrap.
- Freeze until firm.
- Remove from freezer 45 min. to an hour before you wish to serve to give time for fruit cups to thaw enough to thoroughly enjoy.

Vanilla Bean Coconut Yogurt Smoothie

Preparation time: 5 min.
Complete time: 27 min.
Calories 101 – Carbs 5g – Sodium 4g – Fat 9g

What's in it:

- Coconut water (frozen in ice cube tray)
- 1 tsp. torn fresh mint leaves + sprigs for garnishing
- 2 C. Greek yogurt
- 1 vanilla bean (split lengthwise)
- ½ C. honey
- ½ water

How it's made:

- In a saucepan over low heat, combine vanilla bean pod, honey, and water. Simmer for 7-9 min. to allow time for vanilla to infuse into honey. Remove vanilla bean pod and allow time for the mixture to cool completely.
- Combine some of the vanilla honey with yogurt, mint and ½ tray of coconut water in a blender. Blend until smooth in texture.
- Put mixture into glasses. Garnish with a sprig of mint. Serve cold!

Almond-Honey Power Bar

Preparation time: 30 min.
Complete time: 1 hour
Calories 246 – Carbs 38g – Sodium 57mg – Fat 10g

What's in it:

- 1/8 tsp. salt
- ¼ C. honey
- ½ tsp. vanilla extract
- ¼ C. turbinado sugar
- ¼ C. creamy almond butter
- 1/3 C. golden raisins
- 1/3 C. currants
- 1/3 C. dried apricots
- 1 C. unsweetened whole-grain puffed cereal
- 1 tbsp. sesame seeds
- 1 tbsp. flax seeds
- ¼ C. slivered almonds
- ¼ C. unsalted sunflower seeds
- 1 C. old-fashioned rolled oats

How it's made:

- Ensure oven is preheated to 350 degrees. With cooking spray, grease an 8" square pan.
- On a baking sheet with a rim, spread out sesame seeds, flaxseeds, sunflower seeds, almonds, and oats. Bake about 10 min. until oats are just toasted and nuts are fragrant.

Pour in large bowl and add raisins, apricots, currants, and cereal. Toss to ensure thorough combination.
- In a small saucepan, mix together salt, vanilla, honey sugar and almond butter on low heat, ensuring to constantly stir. Perform this action 2 to 5 min. until mixture starts to bubble.
- Quickly pour almond butter batter into dry components, stirring to ensure there are no more visible lumps. Transfer to pan.
- Coat your hands with greasing medium of choice and press mixture into an even layer. Frost for 30 min. or until firm. Cut into 8 bars. Enjoy!

ORANGE RESOLUTION SMOOTHIE

Time: 5 min.
Calories 109 – Carbs 12g – Sodium 98mg – Fat 3g

What's in it:

- 1 banana
- ¼ C. honey
- 1 C. pineapple chunks
- 1 C. orange juice
- 1 C. mini carrots
- 2 C. Greek yogurt
- 2 C. frozen peach slices
- 2 C. frozen mango chunks

How it's made:

- Add all the above components into a blender.
- Blender on high until the consistency comes out creamy and smooth. Enjoy!

Creamy Kale And Eggs

Time: 25 min.
Calories 190 – Carbs 14g – Sodium 213mg – Fat 7g

What's in it:

- 4 slices of toasted crusty bread
- 2 tbsp. grated Parmesan
- 4 large eggs
- ¼ C. 2% Greek yogurt
- Pepper and salt
- Pinch of grated nutmeg
- 1 bunch of kale (stems remove and cut crosswise into thin ribbons)
- 2 tbsp. chopped leeks (both white and green parts)
- 1 tbsp. extra-virgin olive oil

How it's made:

- In a pan over intermediate to immense warmth, warm up oil. Pour in leeks and decrease warmth to low. Cook leeks 8 min. until softened but not browned.
- Pour in kale with leeks and cook 2 min. until wilted. Sprinkle with salt, pepper, and nutmeg to season. Then mix in yogurt. Combine well.

- Make four indentations in the kale and crack an egg into each one. Top each egg with pepper and salt to season.
- Top pan and cook 2 to 3 min. until egg whites are firm and eggs are cooked to the doneness you desire.
- Dive eggs and kale among 4 plates and top with parmesan cheese. Serve with crusty toasted bread.

LUNCH RECIPES

GRILLED SWEET POTATO AND SCALLION SALAD

Preparation time: 10 min.
Complete time: 1 hour
Calories 151 – Carbs 5g – Sodium 4g – Fat 14g

What's in it:

- ¼ C. fresh, roughly cut up parsley
- Pepper and salt
- 1 tsp. honey
- 1 tbsp. balsamic vinegar
- 2 tbsp. apple cider vinegar
- 2 tbsp. Dijon mustard
- 2/3 C. extra-virgin olive oil
- 8 scallions
- 4 large sweet potatoes

How it's made:

- Ensure oven is preheated to 375 degrees. Bake potatoes for 45 min. until softened. Let cool a bit before cutting into large chunks.
- Preheat a grill on high heat. Brush sweet potatoes and scallions with 1/3 cup olive oil.

- Arrange them on grill and grill until they are tender, which takes around 5 min. Remove from grill and cut scallions into smaller pieces.
- Whisk remaining olive oil with mustard, honey, and vinegar, seasoning with pepper and salt. Put in the potatoes, parsley, and scallions into this mixture and gently toss until everything is well coated.

Israeli Couscous Tabouli

Preparation time: 20 min.
Complete time: 28 min.
Calories 180 – Carbs 11g – Sodium 9.8g – Fat 13g

What's in it:

- 3 chopped scallions
- 2 ripe, seeded/diced tomatoes
- 2 tbsp. freshly chopped mint
- ½ C. freshly chopped cilantro
- 1 C. finely chopped parsley
- 3 tbsp. olive oil
- 1 zested and juiced lemon
- Pepper and salt
- 1 C. Israeli couscous

How it's made:

- Over intermediate warmth, pour water in a pot, sprinkle with salt and warm up to a boiling point.
- Pour in couscous and cook it until al dente, around 7 to 8 min. Remove liquid from couscous and set to the side to allow time to cool off a bit.
- Mix together olive oil and lemon juice/zest to create a vinaigrette. Sprinkle pepper and salt if needed to adequately season.

- Mix together scallions, tomatoes, mint, cilantro, parsley and couscous until combined. Toss everything with vinaigrette, seasoning with pepper and salt to achieve desired taste.
- Let the mixture to sit 30 min. so that their flavors can marry together before sitting down and consuming!

Frittata With Asparagus, Tomato, And Fontina

Preparation time: 15 min.
Complete time: 27 min.
Calories 230 – Carbs 11g – Sodium 9g – Fat 12g

What's in it:

- 3 ounces of diced Fontina
- Salt
- 1 seeded/diced tomato
- 12-ounces asparagus (trimmed/cut into ¼-1/2" pieces)
- 1 tbsp. butter
- 1 tbsp. olive oil
- ¼ tsp. pepper
- ½ tsp. salt
- 2 tbsp. whipping cream
- 6 large eggs

How it's made:

- Ensure that your broiler is preheated.
- Whisk together salt, pepper, cream, and eggs.
- In an ovenproof skillet, warm up butter on intermediate to immense warmth.
- Pour in asparagus, sautéing about 2 min. until pieces are crisp-tender.

- Raise heat to intermediate and add in the egg mixture onto asparagus, cooking for a bit to allow eggs to set.
- Top with cheese and decrease heat to medium or low, cooking frittata until set but the top is runny.
- Put the skillet into the broiler. Cook for 5 min. until the top of frittata is firmed and golden in color. Let stand 2 min. before removing from skillet.

Un-Fried Chicken

Preparation time: 10 min.
Complete time: 55 min.
Calories 230 – Carbs 14g – Sodium 10g – Fat – 14g

What's in it:

- 1 ¼ C. cornflake crumbs
- Zest and juice from 1 lemon
- 2 egg whites
- ½ tsp. hot sauce
- ¼ C. low-fat buttermilk
- ½ tsp. chicken seasoning (recipe below)
- 8 skinless, boneless chicken thighs (visible fat trimmed off)
- Non-stick cooking spray

Chicken Seasoning:

- 1 C. salt
- ¼ C. garlic powder
- ¼ C. black pepper

How it's made:

- Ensure oven is preheated to 375 degrees. Grease a cast-iron pan with the greasing medium of your choice. Put over intermediate to immense warmth.
- Sprinkle thighs with chicken seasoning.

- Combine lemon juice/zest, egg whites, buttermilk and hot sauce in a large bowl until combined. Toss in chicken, coating thoroughly.
- Pour cornflake crumbs into another bowl. Dip chicken into these crumbs, pressing gently so that they adhere to chicken.
- Then place chicken in skillet and pop in the oven.
- Back forty to forty-five min. until chicken is golden and a device that reads meat temperature reads 165 degrees or higher.

CHICKEN AND RICE PAPRIKASH CASSEROLE

Preparation time: 10 min.
Complete time: An hour and 50 min.
Calories 311 – Carbs 12g – Sodium 10g – Fat 15g

What's in it:

- 6 tbsp. decreased-fat sour cream
- 2 tbsp. chopped flat-leaf parsley
- 3 C. frozen brown rice (thawed)
- 2 C. low-sodium chicken broth
- 2 tbsp. tomato paste
- 1 tsp. hot paprika or ¼ tsp. cayenne pepper
- 1 tbsp. sweet Hungarian paprika
- 2 large finely chopped red bell peppers
- 2 onions, chopped
- 5 finely chopped cloves of garlic
- 1 tsp. extra virgin olive oil
- Pepper and salt
- 2 pounds of bone-in, skinless chicken thighs

How it's made:

- Ensure oven is preheated to 350 degrees. Pour chicken in a ceramic baking dish. Season with pepper and salt. Bake twenty-five to thirty min., until chicken is just cooked.
- While chicken is cooking, in a saucepan, warm up oil and add in salt, ¼ teaspoon salt,

bell peppers, onions, and garlic. Cook 15 min., mixing around every once in a while until veggies are tender. If mixture becomes too dry, do not be afraid to add a tablespoon or two of water.
- Stir in sweet and hot paprika, cooking for 1 minute. Pour in tomato paste and cook for an additional minute.
- Put chicken broth and 2 cups of water into the pan. Rise up to boiling point, reducing warmth so that a nice simmer is maintained.
- Simmer mixture 5 min. until it becomes thickened.
- Put chicken on a plate and spread rice into the bottom of a dish meant to cook casseroles, topping with chicken and all the juices that it accumulated while cooking.
- Bake 40 min. until casserole is browned on the top.
- Top with parsley and serve alongside a nice dollop of sour cream if you so choose.

TROPICAL CHICKEN PATTIES

Preparation time: 15 min.
Complete time: 40 min.
Calories 517 – Carbs 56g – Sodium 219g – Fat 6g

What's in it:

- ¼ C. chopped fresh cilantro
- 1 ½ C. diced pineapple
- 1 C. frozen peas (thawed)
- 1 C. long grained white rice
- ¼ tsp. turmeric
- 1 finely chopped small red onion
- 2 ½ tbsp. vegetable oil
- Pepper and salt
- ½ tsp. ground allspice
- 2 minced cloves of garlic
- 2 small jalapeño peppers (1 green/1 red – seeded/diced)
- 1 ¼ pounds ground chicken

How it's made:

- In a large bowl, mix up chicken, half of the jalapeño, half the garlic, allspice, ¼ teaspoon salt and ¼ teaspoon pepper until combined.
- Then create four ½" patties. Put patties on a plate and placed covered in the fridge until you are ready to cook them.

- In a large skillet over medium heat, heat up 1 tablespoon vegetable oil. Pour in half the red onion, remaining jalapeño and garlic and turmeric. Cook for 1 minute.
- Add the rice, ¼ teaspoon salt and 2 cups of water. Bring this to a boil.
- Decrease heat to medium-low. Cover and simmer for 15 min. until rice is tender. Add in the peas but cease to stir. Cover and set to the side.
- In a non-stick skillet over intermediate to immense warmth, heat up 1 tablespoon of oil. Add the patties to oil and cook for 4 min. on each side.
- Tin a bowl, toss pineapple cilantro, red jalapeño, remaining red onion and ½ tablespoon vegetable oil. Season with pepper and salt.
- Stir rice and peas and then season with pepper and salt to taste.
- Serve with patties and pineapple salsa.

Healthy Summer Pasta Salad

Preparation time: 25 min.
Complete time: 40 min.
Calories 207 – Carbs 11g – Sodium 11.4g – Fat 8g

What's in it:

- 1 zucchini (cut into small pieces)
- 1 ear of corn (husked and kernels cut from cob)
- 2 tbsp. chopped dill or fresh chives
- 1 C. cherry or grape tomatoes (halved and quartered)
- Pepper and salt, to taste
- ¾ tsp. dry mustard
- 1 ½ tsp. sugar
- 1 ½ tbsp. cider vinegar
- 3 tbsp. sour cream
- ½ C. mayo
- ¼ of one red onion (diced)
- 8 ounces dry cavatappi

How's it made:

- In a large pot, bring salted water to a boil. Add in cavatappi and cook it according to the package. Remove liquid and rinse in cold water. Set to the side.
- While cavatappi is cooking, soak onion in cold water for 5 min. and remove liquid.

- In a bowl, whisk together salt, pepper, remove liquidated red onion, mustard, sugar, oil, vinegar, sour cream and may until combined.
- Pour in zucchini, corn, dill, tomatoes and cooked cavatappi into the dressing. Stir well to coat everything thoroughly. Enjoy!

Chicken Peanut Stir-Fry

Preparation time: 15 min.
Complete time: 25 min.
Calories 476 – Carbs 48g – Sodium 315mg – Fat 14g

What's in it:

- ¼ C. roasted salted peanuts
- 1 small head of Napa cabbage (cored/cut into 2" pieces)
- 1 jalapeño pepper (seeded/thinly sliced)
- 1 bunch of scallions
- One 2" piece of ginger
- 2 tbsp. peanut or vegetable oil
- 1 pound skinless and boneless chicken breasts
- 1 tbsp + 1 tsp. rice vinegar
- 1 tbsp. + 2 tsp. cornstarch
- 3 tsp. soy sauce
- 1 C. basmati rice

How it's made:

- Cook rice according to directions.
- As rice cooks, whisk together 2 teaspoons soy cause and a tablespoon cornstarch and rice vinegar. Pour in chicken and thoroughly coat all sides.
- Mix together remaining cornstarch, 1/3 cup of water, brown sugar and 1 teaspoon soy sauce/rice vinegar in another bowl.

- In a large skillet over immense warmth, warm up a tablespoon of peanut oil. Pour in chicken and stir-fry 2 to 3 min. until lightly golden in color. Remove with slotted spoon to a bowl that is clean.
- Clean out the pan, return to high heat and pour in the peanut oil that remains. When it starts to smoke, add jalapeño, scallion whites, and ginger, stir-frying for 45 seconds to 1 minute. Add in cabbage, stir-frying for three to five min. just until crispy yet tender. Mix in brown sugar mixture and add with chicken. Stir-fry the sauce for 1-2 min. until it is thick and chicken is cooked all the way through.
- Mix in peanuts and scallion greens.
- Serve alongside rice.

Kale And Turkey Rice Bowl

Preparation time: 15 min.
Complete time: 40 min.
Calories 119 – Carbs 13g – Sodium 175mg – Fat 3g

What's in it:

- 2 ½ C. cooked white or brown rice
- One 5 oz. package of chopped kale (6 packed cups)
- ½ pound red skinned potatoes (cut into ½" pieces)
- 1 tsp. ground cumin
- 2 finely chopped cloves garlic
- 1 finely chopped onion
- 1 pound 93% lean ground turkey
- 1 tbsp. vegetable oil
- Salt
- 3 tbsp. sliced almonds
- 1 jalapeño pepper (halved and seeds removed)
- 1 bunch of cilantro (tough stems removed)

How it's made:

- In a blender, puree 3 tablespoons cilantro, ½ cup of water, jalapeño, almonds and ¼ teaspoon of salt until smooth in texture.
- In a large pot or Dutch oven over intermediate to immense warmth, heat

vegetable oil. Add in turkey and ½ teaspoon of salt. Cook for 4 min., stirring to break up turkey with a wooden spoon. Cook until browned.
- Add cumin, garlic, and onion to meat, stirring occasionally until softened. Then pour in 1 ½ cups of water, pureed cilantro mixture, potatoes, and kale. Cover and bring to a boil.
- Uncover and decrease heat to around medium. Let simmer for 15 min., stirring occasionally until potatoes are tender.
- Seasons with pepper and salt as desired. Serve over rice, garnished with leftover cilantro.

ESCAROLE WITH PANCETTA

Calories 124 – Carbs 5g – Sodium 224mg – Fat 2g

What's in it:

- 3 tbsp. diced pancetta
- 2 tbsp olive oil
- 4 garlic cloves
- 1 head chopped escarole

How it's made:

- Cool pancetta until crispy, remove liquid on a paper towel.
- In a skillet cook olive oil and smashed garlic cloves for 1 minute.
- Then add chopped escarole to the pan, cooking for 5 min. until wilted.
- Add pancetta to escarole in a serving dish and season with pepper.

SNACK AND SIDE RECIPES

ROASTED SWEET POTATOES WITH HONEY AND CINNAMON

Preparation time: 15 min.
Complete time: 45 min.
Calories 143 – Carbs 11g – Sodium 7g – Fat 23g

What's in it:

- Pepper and salt, to taste
- 2 tsp. ground cinnamon
- ¼ C. honey
- ¼ C. extra-virgin olive oil + more for drizzling onto cooked potatoes
- 4 sweet potatoes (peeled and cut into 1" cubes)

How it's made:

- Ensure oven is preheated to 375 degrees.
- In a roasting tray, lay out sweet potato cubes. Shower them in oil and honey and then top them with cinnamon, pepper, and salt.
- Roast 25 to 30 min. until tender.

Pull out from the oven and pour onto a serving platter. Drizzle with additional olive oil before serving.

Garlic Mashed Cauliflower

Preparation time: 10 min.
Complete time: 20 min.

What's in it:

- Freshly chopped rosemary, for garnish
- Freshly ground black pepper
- 1 smashed and chopped small clove of garlic
- 1 tbsp. non-fat Greek yogurt
- 1 tbsp. extra-virgin olive oil
- 2 tbsp. grated Parmesan cheese
- ¼ C. chicken stock
- Salt
- 1 medium head of cauliflower, chopped

How it's made:

- In a big pot, raise water up to the point of boiling. Pour in chopped cauliflower and salt. Cook cauliflower 10 min. until it's tenderized.
- Allow time to remove liquid and then dry with a paper towel.
- In a food processor, pour in hot cauliflower with chicken stock, garlic, yogurt, olive oil, and cheese. Process components until they are smooth in texture.
- Stir in a dash of pepper and salt if needed. Proceed in adding in chopped rosemary. Serve!

Strawberry Oatmeal Bars

Preparation time: 10 min.
Complete time: An hour and 20 min.

Calories 136 – Carbs 18g – Sodium 9g – Fat 8.9g

What's in it:

- 1 10-12-ounce jar of strawberry preserves
- ½ tsp. salt
- 1 tsp. baking powder
- 1 C. packed brown sugar
- 1 ½ C. rolled oats
- 1 ½ C. regular white baking flour
- 1 ¾ sticks of unsalted butter (cut into pieces)

How it's made:

- Ensure oven is preheated to 350 degrees. Butter up a rectangular pan.
- Mix salt, baking powder, brown sugar, oat, flour, and butter together until combined.
- Press half of the oat mixture into pan. Then lay out the strawberry preserves over it.
- Top the other half of oat mixture over preserve layer and pat down gently.
- Bake 30 to 40 min. until light brown in color.
- Let cool completely before cutting them into squares.

Fresh Corn Salad

Preparation time: 10 min.
Complete time: 13 min.
Calories 134 – Carbs 6g – Sodium 3g – Fat 9g

What's in it:

- ½ C. julienned fresh basil leaves
- ½ tsp. black pepper
- ½ tsp. salt
- 3 tbsp. olive oil
- 3 tbsp. cider vinegar
- ½ C. small-diced red onion
- 5 ears of shucked corn

How it's made:

- Warm a salted pot of water up to a boil over immense warmth, cooking up corn for 3 min. to decrease starchiness. Remove liquid. Then pour into ice water to stop cooking in order to set the bright, yellow color.
- Once corn is cooled, cut kernels from the cob.
- Pour kernels into onions, salt, pepper, vinegar, and oil of olive in a big bowl. Before eating, mix with fresh basil. Sprinkle with seasonings of choice until you reach desired taste.
- Serve at room temperature or cold.

Kale Chips

Preparation time: 10 min.
Complete time: 1 hour and 25 min.
Calories 17 – Carbs 1g – Sodium .9g – Fat 0g

What's in it:

- Salt
- 1 tsp. za'atar spice
- 1 tsp. dried Mexican oregano
- Olive oil
- 10 kale leaves (washed, dried, stems discarded)

How it's made:

- Ensure oven is preheated to 225 degrees.
- Pour leaves of kale into a bowl and lightly put olive oil over kale until leaves are thoroughly coated and glistening.
- Sprinkle oregano and za'atar over the top of kale. Season with salt and toss gently.
- Transfer kale to baking sheet. Back 45 min. – 1 hour until crispy. Let cool before serving.

Pomegranate Quinoa Pilaf

Preparation time: 15 min.
Complete time: 45 min.
Calories 248 – Carbs 27g – Sodium 89mg - Fat 1g

What's in it:

- ½ C. toasted slivered almonds
- Pepper and salt
- 1 tsp. sugar
- 1 tsp. fresh lemon zest
- ½ a lemon's juice
- 1 tbsp. flat leaf parsley, chopped
- ½ C. scallions (diagonally sliced)
- ½ C. pomegranate seeds
- 2 C. low-sodium chicken broth
- 1 C. quinoa
- ½ medium onion (diced)
- 2 tbsp. olive oil

How it's made:

- In a pan over intermediate to immense warmth, warm up a tablespoon of oil. Sauté the onion until translucent in color and fragrant. Pour in your quinoa and mix to ensure an even coating.
- Add chicken broth and warm up over immense warmth until it reaches the point of boiling. Decrease warmth and simmer twenty

- min. until liquid is quinoa soaks up liquid and is nice and tender.
- Mix together sugar, lemon juice, lemon zest, parsley, scallions, pomegranate seeds and oil until combined. Pour in quinoa and sprinkle with pepper and salt to season until you reach desired taste.
- Garnish with toasted slivered almonds.

Healthy Cauliflower Rice

Preparation time: 10 min.
Complete time: 25 min.
Calories 189 – Carbs 14g – Sodium 27g – Fat 2g

What's in it:

- Juice of ½ lemon
- 2 tbsp. finely chopped parsley leaves
- Salt
- 1 finely diced medium onion
- 3 tbsp. olive oil
- A head of cauliflower

How it's made:

- Trim cauliflower florets, cutting as much of the stem off as possible. Break up florets and pulse in 3 batches in a food processor until mixture is similar to couscous.
- Within a pan over intermediate to immense warmth, warm up oil. As the oil just begins to smoke a bit, add onions, stirring to coat. Cooking onions for 8 min., stirring constantly, until they are golden brown on the edges and soft in texture.
- Add cauliflower, combining well. Then add 1 teaspoon of salt and cook 3 to 5 min. until cauliflower is tender. Take way from the heat.

- In a large serving bowl pour in cauliflower. Garnish with parsley, lemon juice and pepper and salt. Serve warm!

Vanilla Almonds

Preparation time: 5 min.
Complete time: 55 min.
Calories 25 – Carbs 12g – Sodium 12g – Fat 9g

What's in it:

- ½ tsp. ground cinnamon
- ¼ tsp. salt
- ¾ C. sugar
- 4 C. whole almonds
- 1 tsp. pure vanilla extract
- 1 beaten egg white

How it's made:

- Ensure oven is preheated to 300 degrees.
- Mix egg white with vanilla extract, then pour in almonds and stir to ensure even coatings.
- Combine cinnamon, salt, and sugar. Then add to egg white mixture, stirring together well.
- Pour mixture into solitary layer onto a sheet meant for baking that has been liberally greased.
- Bake 20 min.
- Take out of the oven and let cool on waxed paper and then tear into clusters.

WATERMELON AND CUCUMBER SMOOTHIE

Time: 5 min.
Calories 98 – Carbs 10g – Sodium 3g – Fat 0.5g

What's in it:

- 2 C. cubed seedless watermelon (frozen)
- Juice of half a lime (1 tbsp.)
- 1 tbsp. honey (optional)
- 3 tbsp. low-fat buttermilk
- One 2" piece English cucumber (peeled/chopped)

How it's made:

- In a blender, blend honey, lime juice, buttermilk, and cucumber on high until smooth in texture.
- Add half of the frozen watermelon and blend until smooth and well combined. Push down components with a soon before adding in remaining watermelon. Blend until entirety of mix is smooth. Add 1 to 2 tablespoons water if you need to so that you are able to get the right consistency.
- Put into a glass garnished with a cucumber slice.

Slow Cooker Spiced Nuts

Preparation time: 5 min.
Complete time: 4 hours and 5 min.
Calories 89 – Carbs 9g – Sodium 349mg – Fat 9g

What's in it:

- 2 C. unsalted roasted cashews
- 2 C. raw pecans
- 1/8 tsp. cayenne pepper
- 1 tsp. salt
- 2 tsp. orange zest
- 2 tsp. cinnamon
- 3 tbsp. melted unsalted butter
- ¼ C. pure maple syrup

How it's made:

- Line a 6-quart slow cooker with heavy duty foil and liberally grease with greasing medium of choice. Set aside.
- Mix together cayenne, salt, orange zest, cinnamon, butter and maple syrup. Add nuts to the bowl and toss gently to coat thoroughly.
- Pour nuts into the slow cooker in a nice even layer, cover and turn to high.
- Cook for an hour until light syrup forms at the bottom.

- Decrease the warmth to low, stir nuts and cook for another hour, mixing up about every 20 min.
- Turn slow cooker off, uncover and let nuts harder for 2 hours, stirring occasionally.
- Nuts can be stored for 5 days if you do not enjoy right away.

Spicy Summer Squash With Herbs

Preparation time: 10 min.
Complete time: 25 min.
Calories 101 – Carbs 12g – Sodium 201mg – Fat 5g

What's in it:

- ¼ C. minced fresh chives
- 1 minced clove of garlic
- 2 tsp. finely chopped fresh sage or rosemary
- Pepper and salt
- 1 ½ tsp. white wine vinegar
- 1 diced onion
- 1 minced small jalapeño (leave some seeds within)
- 3 medium yellow or green summer squash (diced)
- 1 ½ tbsp. extra-virgin olive oil

How it's made:

- Within a pan on intermediate to immense warmth, warm up oil. Pour in pepper and salt, vinegar, onions, jalapeños, and squash, stirring to combine. Cover and cook 6 min. until squash starts to become brown in color.
- Remove lid and continue cooking process for another 6 min. until squash is browned nicely. Add sage and garlic and cook for

another minute. Sprinkle with pepper and salt to season in order to achieve desired taste.

- Stir in chives. Pour into a bowl and serve!

Pumpkin-Parmesan Biscuits

Preparation time: 30 min.
Complete time: 50 min.
Calories 105 – Carbs 12g – Sodium 200mg – Fat 5g

What's in it:

- ¼ C. heavy cream
- ½ C. canned pure pumpkin
- 1 stick cold unsalted butter + more for brushing (diced)
- 2 tbsp. finely grated parmesan cheese
- ¼ tsp. freshly grated nutmeg
- 1 tsp. salt
- 1 tbsp. sugar
- 1 tbsp. baking powder
- 2 C. all-purpose flour + more for dusting

How it's made:

- Ensure oven is preheated to 400 degrees. With parchment paper, line a sheet in which you can bake on.
- Mix nutmeg, salt, sugar baking powder, and flour together. Then add in 1 tablespoon of parmesan. Add in diced butter and with the mixture with fingertips until it resembles coarse crumbs.
- In a separate bowl, mix cream and pumpkin together and put over flour mixture. Mix

with hands or a fork to create a softened dough.
- Put dough on a flat surface that has been mildly floured. Roll out into ¾" thick rectangle using a floured rolling pin.
- Cut out biscuits and arrange them on the baking sheet about 2" apart. Pour a bit of nicely melted butter over the tops before sprinkling with remaining parmesan.
- Bake 15 - 20 min. until biscuits are richly colored.
- Let sit on a rack made of wire to cool. Allow cooling a bit before serving.

POTATOES WITH CHILI BUTTER

Preparation time: 5 min.
Complete time: 25 min.
Calories 165 – Carbs 20g – Sodium 174mg – Fat 9g

What's in it:

- 1 pound of new potatoes
- ½ tsp. chili powder
- 3 tbsp. butter
- Pepper and salt

How it's made:

- In a pot of cold salted water, add one pound of new potatoes. Warm up to the point of boiling and cook fifteen to twenty min. until potatoes become tenderized. Remove liquid them.
- In a pan, melt 3 tablespoons of butter and add ½ teaspoon of chili powder as well as a sprinkle or two of pepper and salt to season.
- Drizzle chili butter over potatoes. A great side!

Tomato Gratin

Preparation time: 4 min.
Complete time: 15 min.
Calories 109 – Carbs 12g – Sodium 123mg – Fat 2g

What's in it:

- 2 pints of grape tomatoes
- 4 garlic cloves
- ¼ C. olive oil
- 2 tsp. fresh thyme
- ½ C. parmesan
- ½ C. breadcrumbs

How it's made:

- In an ovenproof skillet over intermediate to immense warmth, cook grape tomatoes, smash garlic cloves, ¼ cup of olive oil and thyme for 8 min. until tomatoes are softened.
- Within the means of a bowl, mix remaining olive oil, breadcrumbs, and parmesan together.
- Sprinkle parmesan mixture over tomatoes.
- Broil 3 min. until the dish is a golden brown color.

Eggplant Caponata

Complete Time: 25 min.
Calories 138 – Carbs 14g – Sodium 199mg – Fat 1g

What's in it:

- 1 chopped onion
- ¼ C. olive oil
- 1 stalk of celery, chopped
- 1 eggplant, chopped
- 1 chopped red bell pepper
- 3 tbsp. golden raisins
- 1 tbsp. chopped oregano
- ½ C. water
- 1 C. halved grape tomatoes
- 1 tbsp. cider vinegar
- 1 tbsp. capers
- Pepper and salt, to taste
- Torn basil, for garnish

How it's made:

- In a pan, cook onion alongside olive oil 3 min. Then pour in celery and eggplant and cook an additional 4 min.
- Pour in red bell pepper, cooking for 3 min. Then pour in raisins, oregano, and water. Bubble for eight min.
- Pour in capers, apple cider vinegar, and grape tomatoes. Cook for 7 min.

- Sprinkle with pepper and salt to season in order to achieve desired taste and garnish with basil before serving.

Italian Lentil Salad

Preparation time: 8 min.
Complete time: 28 min.
Calories 198 – Carbs 11g – Sodium 89mg – Fat 2g

What's in it:

Salad:

- 2 tsp. lemon zest
- ½ C. coarsely chopped skinned/toasted hazelnuts
- 1 red bell pepper that has been seeded and diced
- 1 cucumber that has been peeled, seeded and diced
- 1 C. seedless red grapes that have been cut in half
- 1 C. seedless green grapes that have been cut in half
- 2 scallions, cut up
- 1 pound green lentils (Sabarot recommended)

Vinaigrette:

- ¼ tsp. ground black pepper
- ½ tsp. salt
- 1/3 C. extra-virgin olive oil
- 1/3 C. fresh lemon juice

How it's made:

- *For the salad*: Get out a pot. Pour in water and salt and warm up liquid up to the point of boiling. Pour in lentils and cook 18 - 20 min. until tenderized, ensuring to stir periodically. Remove liquid. Let cool off for 5 min. at the very least.
- Pour lentils and remaining salad components into a large salad bowl.
- *For vinaigrette:* In a small bowl, pour in lemon juice. Gradually add in oil, mixing rapidly until incorporated. Sprinkle with pepper and salt to season in order to achieve desired taste. Enjoy!

DINNER RECIPES

Oven Baked Salmon

Preparation time: 5 min.
Complete time: 20 min.
Calories 290 – Carbs 17g – Sodium 11g – Fat 9g

What's in it:

- 12-ounce salmon fillet
- Coarse salt
- Black pepper
- Toasted almond parsley salad (for serving)
- Baked squash (optional: for serving)

Toasted Almond Parsley Salad

- Extra-virgin olive oil
- ½ C. toasted almonds
- 1 C. flat-leaf parsley
- 2 tbsp. rinsed capers
- Coarse salt
- 1 tbsp. red wine vinegar
- 1 shallot

How it's made:

- Ensure oven is preheated to 450 degrees.

- Sprinkle fillets of salmon with pepper and salt to season.
- Put salmon on a baking sheet, with the skin side touching the pan, preferably non-stick.
- Bake twelve to fifteen min. until salmon is cooked all the way through.
- Serve with toasted almond parsley salad if you desire!

Toasted Almond Parsley Salad:

- Slice and dice shallot then pour vinegar over shallots, adding a pinch of salt to season. Allow time for the mixture to sit for 30 min.
- Cut up almonds, capers, and parsley, adding to shallots. Pour in olive oil to taste. Mix and adjust seasonings as needed.

Pork Tenderloin With Seasoned Rub

Preparation time: 5 min.
Complete time: 35 min.
Calories 310 – Carbs 29g – Sodium 10g – Fat 18g

What's in it:

- 1 tsp. minced garlic
- 1 tbsp. olive oil
- 1 ¼ pounds of pork tenderloin
- Salt, to taste
- 1 tsp. dried thyme
- 1 tsp. ground coriander
- 1 tsp. ground cumin
- 1 tsp. dried oregano
- 1 tsp. garlic powder

How it's made:

- Ensure oven is preheated to 450 degrees.
- Mix all dry components until well incorporated. This is the rub for your tenderloin.
- Sprinkle rub over tenderloin and proceed to rub into all sides of meat.
- Pour olive oil in a pan over intermediate to immense warmth. Pour in garlic and proceed to sauté for a minute, stirring constantly.
- Place tenderloin in the pan, cooking 10 min. per side, turning meat with tongs.

- Upon a nice roasting pan, place your meat and bake 20 min.
- Cut, serve and enjoy!

Mushroom Stuffer Pork Tenderloin

Preparation Time: 25 min.
Complete time: 1 hour and 10 min.
Calories 290 – Carbs 12g – Sodium 13g – Fat 23g

What's in it:

- ½ tsp. grated lemon zest
- 2 pork tenderloins
- ½ C. chopped fresh parsley
- 1 tbsp. breadcrumbs
- 1 clove of garlic
- Pepper and salt
- 8 ounces of thinly sliced cremini mushrooms
- 4 slices chopped low-sodium bacon
- 5 tbsp. extra virgin olive oil + extra for basting

How it's made:

- In a large pan over intermediate to immense warmth, warm up 2 tablespoons of oil. Pour in bacon and cook about eight min. until nice and crispy.
- Pour in mushrooms, ½ tsp. pepper and salt and cook mushrooms until soft.
- Pour in garlic and cook for a minute.
- Take pan away from heat and mix in breadcrumbs and all but a couple

tablespoons of parsley until combined. Set aside to cool.
- Immerse ten to twelve toothpicks in liquid to avoid burning them in the oven later. Rinse off meat and then dry graciously. Butterfly cut the tenderloin, cutting it like a book so that meat ends up lying flat.
- Cover pork in a wrap made of plastic and beat with a meat hammer until it is ½" thick.
- Spread mushroom mixture over tenderloins and secure the seams with soaked toothpicks.
- Preheat grill on intermediate to immense warmth, brushing the grates with olive oil. Brush pork rolls with oil and season with pepper and salt.
- Grill tenderloins, turning frequently until a thermometer says 140 degrees. Transfer to a cutting board and let rest for 10 min.
- Mix up remaining olive oil and parsley with lemon zest, pepper, and salt. Remove toothpicks from meat and slice pork rolls. Top with parsley oil and serve.

Four-Step Lemon-Onion Chicken

Preparation time: 15 min.
Complete time: 40 min.
Calories 467 –Carbs 16g – Sodium 282mg – Fat 6g

What's in it:

- 4 boneless, skinless chicken breast halves (sliced in half horizontally)
- 1 9-ounce bag spinach
- Juice of 2 lemons
- 1 C. low-sodium chicken broth
- ¼ C. white wine (optional)
- 1 small bunch of fresh thyme leaves (chopped)
- 1 thinly sliced red onion
- ¼ C. all-purpose flour
- 3 tbsp. extra-virgin olive oil
- Pepper and salt, to taste
- 1 tsp. dried thyme

How it's made:

- Season chicken with thyme, pepper, and salt.
- In a large sauté pan over intermediate to immense warmth, heat olive oil.
- Put flour in a shallow dish and dredge chicken in batches.

- Adding chicken to pan, sauté on both sides for 3 min. per side. Transfer to plate and cover with foil.
- Add red onion and thyme to the pan and cook over low heat for 5 min., stirring every now and again until aromatic.
- Combine wine, chicken broth and lemon juice in a bowl. Turn heat up to high and deglaze broth mixture, scraping the pan with wooden spoon.
- Cook for about 10 min. until liquid starts to decrease. Remove from heat and whisk in 1 ½ tablespoons butter. Season with pepper and salt.
- Put spinach in a microwave-safe bowl and add 3 tablespoons water, covering loosely with plastic wrap. Microwave 5-6 min. until wilted.
- Remove liquid and toss with remaining butter, juice of other lemon and salt/pepper to taste.
- Arrange on serving platter on top of chicken. Spoon sauce over the top and serve!

Dry Rubbed London Broil

Preparation time: 8 min.
Complete time: 23 min.
Calories 219 – Carbs 12g – Sodium 110mg – Fat 11.8g

What's in it:

- 2 tbsp. olive oil
- One 2 pound London broil
- 1 recipe Dave's Rub

Dave's Rub

- 15 grinds black pepper
- 4 pinches salt
- 2 tsp. garlic powder
- 1 tbsp. sweet paprika
- 1 tbsp. dried oregano
- 2 tbsp. chili powder

How it's made:

- Rub London broil with olive oil and generously apply dry rub. Let sit for 15 min. at room temperature.
- Preheat a grill pan on intermediate to immense warmth.
- Place meat on grill and grill for 5 min. per side for medium-rare.

- Remove from heat and let rest for 5-10 min. before slicing.

Herbed Tuna Steaks

Preparation time: 1 hour and 10 min.
Complete time: 1 hour and 20 min.
Calories 198 – Carbs 12g – Sodium 209mg – Fat 9g

What's in it:

- Pepper and salt, to taste
- Two 1-pound center-cut tuna steaks (1" in thickness)
- 3 tbsp. extra-virgin olive oil
- 3 scallions
- 6 sprigs thyme (leaves stripped)
- 3 sprigs rosemary (leaves stripped)

How it's made:

- Roughly chop scallions, thyme, and rosemary and put into a small bowl, mix with a tablespoon of oil.
- Within a shallow dish, season tuna steaks with pepper and salt. Rub with herb mixture on both sides. Cover and Frost for 1-4 hours.
- In a pan on high heat, warm up remaining olive oil. Place tuna in skillet and sear two to three min. on each side until rich in color to achieve medium rare tuna steaks.
- Place on a board meant for cutting for 5 min. to rest before proceeding to slice. Enjoy!

Steamed Shrimp Dumplings

Preparation time: 1 hour
Complete time: 1 hour 40 min.
Calories 234 – Carbs 17g – Sodium 125mg – Fat 6g

What's in it:

- 36 round dumpling wrappers
- Pinch of white pepper
- ½ tsp. sugar
- Salt
- ¾ tsp. toasted sesame oil
- 1 ½ tsp. dry sherry
- 1 ½ tbsp. cornstarch
- 2 finely chopped scallions
- 1/3 C. water chestnuts, cut up finely
- ¾ pound large shrimp (peeled/deveined/chopped finely)
- 1 large egg white

Ponzu dipping sauce:

- 3 tbsp. ponzu sauce
- 1 tsp. soy sauce
- ½ tsp. sesame oil
- 1 chopped scallion

How it's made:

- In a large bowl, beat egg white. Add ¼ teaspoon salt, pepper, sugar, sesame oil, sherry, cornstarch, scallions, chestnuts, and shrimp. Combine well for 1 minute until it starts to thicken. Frost for 1 hour.
- On a clean surface covered with a damp paper towel, set out 1 dumpling wrapper. Stir 1 heaping teaspoon of shrimp mixture into the wrapper. Dab a finger into a bowl of cold water to moisten edges of the wrapper. Fold in half and press together the edges to seal. Place onto a sheet meant for baking. Perform this process with the remainder of dumpling wrappers.
- Fill up a pan with ¼" of water and bring to a boil. Working in batches, add dumplings in a single layer, cover and steam for 5 min. to cook.
- Transfer cooked dumpling to a plate.
- To make dipping sauce: mix all sauce components together in a small bowl until combined. Serve along with dumplings!

BRAISED CHICKEN WITH MUSHROOMS

Preparation time: 20 min.
Complete time: 3 hours and 10 min.
Calories 218 – Carbs 23g – Sodium 319mg – Fat 8g

What's in it:

- ½ C. celery tops or flat-leaf parsley (chopped)
- ½ - ¾ C. white wine
- 2 large bay leaves
- Few sprigs of thyme (finely chopped)
- 5-6 cloves of garlic (thinly sliced)
- 2 ribs celery (finely chopped)
- 2 carrots (finely chopped)
- 2 onions (sliced)
- 1 pound cremini mushrooms (thinly sliced)
- Pepper and salt, to taste
- 4 pieces of chicken leg quarters (Bone-in, skin on)
- Olive oil, for frying
- 2 C. chicken stock
- 1 ounce dried porcini mushrooms

How it's made:

- In a small pot over intermediate to immense warmth, pour in dried mushrooms and stock. Bring to boil and then decrease to low in order to reconstitute.

- In a large skillet with a lid, heat a thin layer of olive oil over intermediate to immense warmth. Pat chicken dry and season liberally with pepper and salt. Brown only half the chicken at a time, skin side down for 5 min. Then turn chicken and cook an additional 3-4 min. on another side.
- Remove browned chicken to a plate and place fresh mushrooms, cooking 10-15 min. Pour in salt, pepper, bay leaves, thyme, garlic, celery, carrot, and onion, stirring and cooking for another 10 min. until softened.
- Deglaze pot with white wine. Add chicken back into the pot and arrange veggies and mushrooms around it. Pour stock over chicken, reserving a few spoonfuls.
- Cover and braise on low, simmering for 30 min. Serve.

Coffee Rubbed Steak With Peppers And Onions

Preparation time: 30 min.
Complete time: 45 min.
Calories 321 – Carbs 23g – Sodium 334mg – Fat 9.8g

What's in it:

- Juice of ½ a lime + lime wedges for garnish
- 1 green bell pepper (cut into strips)
- Ground black pepper
- 1 onion (cut into wedges)
- 2 tsp. vegetable oil
- One 1 ¼ - 1 ½ inch skirt steak (cut into 4 pieces)
- Salt
- 1/8 tsp. ground cinnamon
- ½ tsp. ancho chili powder
- 1 tsp. mustard powder
- 1 tsp. unsweetened cocoa powder
- 1 tbsp. instant coffee
- 2 tbsp. + 1 tsp. pack light or dark brown sugar

How it's made:

- In a bowl, mix together 1 teaspoon salt, cinnamon, chili powder, mustard powder, cocoa powder, instant coffee and 2 tablespoons brown sugar. Rub between fingers until fine in texture. Season steak with salt and generously rub coffee-spice mixture on.

- In a cast-iron skillet over medium heat, heat up vegetable oil. Sear steak 3-6 min. on each side for medium rare. Put onto a cutting board and let rest. Reserve juices from the steak that are in skillet.
- Add remaining brown sugar and onion into the skillet, sprinkling with pepper and salt to taste. Cook on intermediate to immense warmth for 5 min. until onion is golden and soft.
- Then add bell pepper and ¼ cup of water, cooking for 5 min., stirring until crisp yet tender. Stir in lime juice, season with more pepper and salt.
- Slice skirt steak against the grain. Divide bell peppers, onions, and juices from steak among plates. Serve with lime wedges and cornbread.

DESSERT RECIPES

Angel Food Cake

Preparation time: 20 min.
Complete time: 55 min.
Calories 267 – Carbs 12g – Sodium 7g – Fat 13g

What's in it:

- 1 ½ tsp. cream of tartar
- 1 tsp. orange extract
- 1/3 C. warm water
- 12 egg whites (room temperature)
- 1 C. sifted cake flour
- ¼ tsp. salt
- 1 ¾ C. sugar

How it's made:

- Ensure oven is preheated to 350 degrees.
- Spin sugar in a food processor for 2 min. until sugar is super fine in texture.
- Sift half of sugar with salt and cake flour, setting another half aside.
- Whisk cream of tartar, orange extract, water and egg whites in a large bowl. Once you

have whisked for 2 min., switch to a hand mixer.
- Slowly sift in reserved sugar, beating constantly at medium speed.
- When you have achieved medium peaks, sift enough of the flour mixture to dust the top of the foam. Using a spatula, fold gently. Continue to do this until all of the flour mixtures is well incorporated.
- Spoon mixture carefully into an un-greased tube or bundt pan.
- Bake for 35 min. and check for doneness with a wooden skewer.
- Cool upside down on a cooling rack for at least 1 hour before attempting to remove from pan.

Cocoa Brownies

Preparation time: 15 min.
Complete time: 1 hour and 15 min.
Calories 200 – Carbs 11g – Sodium 4g – Fat 8g

What's in it:

- ½ tsp. salt
- ½ C. sifted flour
- 2 tsp. vanilla extract
- 1 ¼ C. sifted cocoa
- 8 ounces melted butter
- 1 C. sifted brown sugar
- 1 C. sifted sugar
- 4 eggs
- Flour, to dust pan
- Soft butter, for greasing pan

How it's made:

- Ensure oven is preheated to 300 degrees.
- Butter and flour an 8" square pan.
- Mix eggs until fluffy and light yellow in color. Then pour in both sugars and remaining components, mixing well until incorporated.
- Put batter into greased pan meant for baking. Bake 45 min. or until toothpick turns out with no more batter on it that has been inserted in the center.

- Once baked, set on a wire rack to allow to adequately cool.

Lemon Ricotta Cookies With Lemon Glaze

Preparation time: 15 min.
Complete time: 2 hours and 50 min.
Calories 149 – Carbs 9g – Sodium 4g – Fat 12g

What's in it:

- 1 zested lemon
- 3 tbsp. lemon juice
- 1 15 oz. container of whole milk ricotta cheese
- 2 eggs
- 2 C. sugar
- 1 stick softened unsalted butter
- 1 tsp. salt
- 1 tsp. baking powder
- 2 ½ C. regular white baking flour

Glaze:

- 1 zested lemon
- 3 tbsp. lemon juice
- 1 ½ C. powdered sugar

How it's made:

- Ensure oven is preheated to 375 degrees.
- Mary together salt, flour, and baking powder.
- In yet another bowl, cream up sugar and butter. With the help of a mixer that you plug

in, combine butter and sugar for three min. until it is fluffy and very lightened in texture. Pour in eggs one at a time, mixing each you're your reach ensured blending. Then pour in ricotta cheese, lemon zest/juice. Beat until combined.

- Mix in dry components.
- Line a couple of baking sheets with parchment paper. Pour cookie dough (2 tbsp. per cookie) onto sheets.
- Bake 15 min. until the edges of the cookies are slightly golden brown. Let cookies rest for 20 min.
- *For glaze:* Stir together lemon zest/juice and powdered sugar until smooth in texture. Spoon ½ teaspoon of glaze onto each cookie using the back of a spoon.
- Allow time for glaze harden (2 hours should be good!) Enjoy!

Espresso Chip Meringues

Calories 23 – Carbs 2g – Sodium .5g – Fat .5g

What's in it:

- 2/3 C. mini semi-sweet chocolate chips
- 2 tsp. instant espresso powder
- ¼ tsp. pure vanilla extract
- 1/8 tsp. cream of tartar
- ¾ C. superfine sugar
- Pinch of fine sea salt
- 3 larger egg whites (room temperature)

How it's made:

- Ensure oven is preheated to 300 degrees. Make sure that the rack that lives within the means of your oven is positioned in the center of your oven before preheating.
- With parchment paper, line a sheet and set to the side.
- Beat egg whites at low speed for a minute until fluffy. A tablespoon at a time, stir in your sugar. Then pour in cream of tartar, vanilla extract, and espresso powder.
- With the help of an electric mixer, beat mixture 3 to 5 min. until it is thick and holds stiff peaks. Fold in chocolate chips.

- Drop ¼-1/2 cupfuls of mixture onto baking sheet, ensuring there are at least 2 inches between each.
- Bake 30 min. Take out of the oven, rotating pan and pop back in the oven to bake another 30 min.
- Turn off oven, allowing meringues to sit in the oven to cool. This should take about 2 hours.
- Take out of the oven and allow time for them to cool down. You can store uneaten ones for up to 4 days in a container that seals well.

HEALTHY NO-BAKE CHOCOLATE PEANUT BUTTER BARS

Preparation time: 10 min.
Complete time: 4 hours and 10 min.
Calories 189 – Carbs 12g – Sodium 109mg – Fat 10g

What's in it:

Crust:

- 4 oz. melted semi-sweet chocolate morsels
- 3 tbsp. melted unsalted butter
- 24 chocolate wafer cookies
- Cooking spray

Filling:

- 2/3 C. confectioners' sugar
- ½ C. 2% Greek yogurt
- ½ C. creamy all-natural peanut butter
- 4 oz. decreased-fat cream cheese

Topping:

- Salt
- ¼ C. chopped unsalted peanuts

How it's made:

- *For crust:* Line an 8" square pan with foil, letting some hang over the side. Lightly coat with cooking spray.
- Process cookies until they are finely ground within the means of a food processor. Pour in melted butter during this process until crumbs are thoroughly coated with butter.
- Add in melted chocolate morsels and process until mixture resembles a wet sand texture.
- Press cookie mixture into bottom of the prepared pan. Cover and frost when filled. Clean out the food processor.
- *For the filling:* In the cleaned out processor pour in sugar, yogurt, peanut butter, and cream cheese, mixing until creamy and smooth.
- Pour mixture over cookie crust. Top with peanuts and sprinkle with ¼ teaspoon salt.
- Top with a cover and Frost within the means of your refrigerator for at least 4 hours or during the course of the night. Knife into twelve bars and serve!

Greek Yogurt Cheesecake

Preparation time: 20 min.
Complete time: 4 hours and 40 min.
Calories 211 – Carbs 21.1g – Sodium 132mg – Fat 12g

What's in it:

- 1 tsp. unflavored gelatin
- ¾ C. unsweetened pineapple juice
- 2 C. frozen wild blueberries
- Salt
- 1 tsp. lemon zest
- 1 tsp. vanilla extract
- ¼ C. all-purpose flour
- ¾ C. sugar
- 3 large eggs
- 8 ounces decreased-fat cream cheese (room temperature)
- One 17 oz. container of 2% Greek yogurt
- 2 tbsp. melted unsalted butter
- 2 C. slightly crushed cinnamon sugar pita chips

How it's made:

- Ensure oven is preheated to 325 degrees with the oven rack positioned in the center. Coat a 9" springform pan with greasing medium of your choice. Wrap sides and bottom of the pan with foil. Place pan on baking sheet.

- In a food processor, pulse pita chips until they are fine. Pour in butter and process until crumbs become moistened.
- Take the crumbs and press into the bottom of the pan, using about ½ of a cup along the sides.
- Bake crust for 5 min. until it looks slightly dry and fragrant.
- In a clean food processor, combine ½ teaspoon salt, lemon zest, vanilla, flour, sugar, eggs, cream cheese and yogurt until all components are smooth and well mixed.
- Add cream cheese mixture to the crust you prepared earlier.
- Bake 40 to 50 min. until middle is set.
- Allow time for the cheesecake to completely.
- Top with a cover and allow to Frost for at least 3 hours or during the course of the night.
- *For topping*: In a saucepan, bring blueberries and pineapple juice to the point of boiling. Decrease the warmth to low and simmer five min. Take away from the heat.
- Pour gelatin and 1 tablespoon of water into a bowl and allow to sit for 5 min. Then proceed to stir dissolved gelatin into hot berry mixture until well mixed. Put this mixture in another bowl and let Frost for at least 3 hours until thickened.

- Once cheesecake is Frosted, take away from the pan. Slice and consume with blueberry sauce topped over the top of the cake.

APPLE AND BERRY BROWN BETTY

Preparation time: 25 min.
Complete time: 1 hour and 10 min.
Calories 290 – Carbs 17g – Sodium 390mg – Fat 11g

What's in it:

- Vanilla ice cream or whipped cream (optional topping)
- ½ tsp. salt
- ½ C. chopped almonds
- ½ C. packed light brown sugar
- 1 C. crushed sugar cones (about 6)
- 2 tbsp. all-purpose flour
- Zest and juice from ½ a lemon
- ½ tsp. nutmeg
- 1 tsp. cinnamon
- 1/3 C. granulated sugar
- 2 C. blackberries
- 4 Golden Delicious Apples
- 1 melted stick of unsalted butter + more for dish

How it's made:

- Ensure oven is preheated to 350 degrees. Butter a 1 ½ quart dish meant for baking.
- In a large vessel that is bowl shaped, toss together 4 tablespoons butter, flour, lemon juice/zest, ¼ teaspoon nutmeg, ½ teaspoon

cinnamon, sugar, blackberries, and apples until everything is coated.
- Combine cones, brown sugar, remaining cinnamon, ¼ teaspoon nutmeg, almonds, salt and remaining butter in another bowl.
- Pour half of apple-berry mixture into prepared dish. Then top mixture with half of the cone mixture. Put remaining apple-berry mixture over top and top with rest of cone mixture.
- Bake 40-45 min. until apples are soft and top is golden brown in color.
- Transfer dish to a rack made of wire and let sit for 10 min. before consuming.
- Serve with ice cream or whipped cream. Yum!

Chewy Gluten Free Chocolate Chip Cookies

Preparation time: 25 min.
Complete time: 1 hour and 39 min.
Calories 119 – Carbs 14g – Sodium 249mg – Fat 7g

What's in it:

- 12 ounces of semisweet chocolate chips
- 1 ½ tsp. vanilla extract
- 1 egg yolk
- 1 whole egg
- 1 ¼ C. packed light brown sugar
- ¼ C. sugar
- 1 tsp. baking soda
- 1 tsp. salt
- 1 tsp. xanthan gum
- 2 tbsp. tapioca flour
- ¼ C. cornstarch
- 2 C. brown rice flour
- 8 oz. unsalted butter

How it's made:

- In a saucepan over low warmth, allow time for the butter to melt. Once liquefied, pour into a stand mixer bowl.
- Sift rice flour, cornstarch, tapioca flour, xanthan gum, salt and baking soda together. Set to the side.

- Add both sugars to stand mixer with liquefied butter. Mix with paddle attachment on intermediate speed for a minute. Pour in the whole egg, egg yolk, vanilla extract and milk, mixing well until thoroughly combined.
- Gradually incorporate flour mixture until mixed well. Then pour in chocolate chips and mix until combined.
- Frost dough in the fridge for at least 1 hour.
- Ensure oven is preheated to 375 degrees. Form your dough into balls that equal about two ounces and put onto a baking sheet prepared with parchment paper. Six cookies should fit on each of your sheets.
- Bake fourteen min., turning pans around after seven min. of bake time.
- Take away from the oven and let cool on a rack made of wire. Indulge!

Jam-And-Oat Squares

Preparation time: 10 min.
Complete time: 25 min.
Calories 210 – Carbs 32g – Sodium 74mg – Fat 4g

What's in it:

- 1 Frosted pie crust
- ¾ C. strawberry jam
- ¾ C. oats
- ¾ C. flour
- 6 tbsp. melted butter
- 1/3 C. packed brown sugar
- ¼ C. granulated sugar
- Pinch of salt

How it's made:

- Ensure oven is preheated to 450 degrees.
- On a baking sheet prepared with parchment paper, unroll pie crust.
- Spread crust with strawberry jam, ensuring that you leave at least a ½" border.
- Mix oat and flour together in a bowl and add melted butter, brown sugar, granulated sugar, and salt. Combine well.
- Squeeze sugar mixture into clumps over jam.
- Bake for 15 min.
- Allow time for them to cool before cutting into desired squares.

CONCLUSION

Thank you for making it through to the end of *Blood Pressure Solution*.

I hope that the contents of this book were able to bring to light a health issue that plagues many individuals and how you can easily correct it and create a healthier you through the means of what you consume!

I hope that this book was informative and able to adequately provide you with all the tools that are necessary to achieve your goals of lowering your blood pressure and reducing hypertension before your next doctor's appointment!

The next step is to get crack-a-lackin'! Pick out which of the delicious recipes you want to try out first and make a grocery list! You will not know the amazing effects that these recipes will have on your life if you never get the initiative to try them out! I assure you, your taste buds will not be disappointed! It is not about sacrificing taste and satisfaction, but using correct ingredient combinations of food in order to help your body minimize the things that lead to heightened blood pressure levels and hypertension within the body.

Once again, don't forget to grab a copy of your FREE BONUS book "Super Foods For Super Health". If you are interested in learning more about the easily accessible super foods that you could incorporate into your diet and transform your overall health, then this book is for you.

Just go to http://bit.ly/superfoods-gift

Good luck my friends! You have made the great decision to embark on a journey that will eventually lead to a healthier you! Over time you will see and feel the difference these recipes will make. And your doctor will too!

THANK YOU!

Before you go, I just wanted to say thank you for purchasing my book.

You could have picked from dozens of other books on the same topic but you took a chance and chose this one.

So, a HUGE thanks to you for getting this book and for reading all the way to the end.

Now I wanted to ask you for a small favor. Could you please take just a few minutes to leave a review for this book on Amazon?

This feedback will help me continue to write the type of books that will help you get the results you want. So if you enjoyed it, please let me know! (-:

Printed in Great Britain
by Amazon